ETHICAL FITNESS

Recipes for eating vegan while getting fit

AMINE SALHI

TABLE OF CONTENTS

Introduction..1

Breakfast...3

   Banana Chocolate Pancakes 3

   Oatmeal with Fruit and Nuts..5

   Breakfast Burrito...7

   Waffles 9

Lunch 11

   Lentil Bowl 11

   Flaxseed Burger 13

   Seed Pizza 15

   Vegetable and Bean Soup 17

   Peppers Stuffed With Quinoa 20

   Chickpea Sandwich With Roasted Sunflower Seeds....................23

   Roasted Pumpkin Soup 26

   Broccoli, Asparagus, Carrot, and Pea Soup...................29

   Spinach, Red Cabbage, and Herb Salad.........................31

   Vinaigrette Pasta Salad 33

   Red Dal 35

Dinner: 37

   Black Bean Baked Potato..37

   Vegetable Pasta...39

   Vegan Lasagna..42

   Stir Fried Noodles 45

Snacks: **48**

Red Pepper Hummus 48

Antioxidant Smoothie 50

Avocado Smoothie 52

Sweet Potato Fries 54

Desserts **56**

Vegan Banana Cream Pie 56

Vegan Brownies 60

INTRODUCTION

What is veganism? Put simply, veganism is a lifestyle choice in which a person makes as little impact on the planet as possible. This is usually done through choosing not to eat meat, not to eat anything made from animal products, not to support any businesses that treat the Earth and its inhabitants unethically, etc. For many vegans this is a choice based on compassion, yet many new vegans are quickly alarmed at how many products use one or more animals products at some stage in their production. Therefore, living this lifestyle takes vigilance and dedication, meaning that books like this are essential to create recipes that are both delicious yet consciousness.

Of course, restricting your diet in any form means that one needs to be aware of what nutrients your body needs and how to get them. When it comes to veganism, because all protein rich animal products have been eliminated, it may be difficult to get enough protein during the day. This is especially true for people with an active lifestyle, such as athletes, whose bodies require substantially more nutrients than the average person. Likewise, some vegans are risk of not getting enough vitamin B12, which is mainly contained in animal products. When a person does not get enough of this essential vitamin, he or she may experience negative effects on their nervous systems, may have a compromised immune system, may develop anemia, among many other side effects. Therefore, this book has focused creating meals that contain high amounts of protein and B12, so that people can create healthy and delicious meals to fuel their fitness based lifestyle.

While some people in society believe that vegans do not get enough nutrition to excel, there are numerous highly productive famous people that prove this wrong. For example, Beyonce announced on Twitter a few years ago that she had given up all animal products. Jessica Chastain, who is the child of a vegan chef, has been going down this path for over a decade. Natalie Portman has been a vegan for most of her life, and, in fact, she believes in it so much that she helped create a famous vegan documentary. Even Mike Tyson converted to veganism for a stint, as he believed it would help cleanse his system of all the drugs and medications that he had been taken, although this was after his physical prime. Famous musician Stevie Wonder also went vegan not to long ago, with him claiming that it has drastically improved his lifestyle.

When it comes to active, world class athletes, several have given up all animal products, yet are still able to perform at the top level. For example, Heather Mills is a professional skier, Scott Jurek is an ultramarathon runner, Meagan Duhamel is a professional figure skater, Patrik Baboumian is a competitive strongman, Alex Morgan is a professional soccer player, among many, many others. Each of these people have chosen to eat an ethical diet, yet these have not compromised their level of nutrition. How do they do this? Well, the answer is understanding how to get everything you need through careful research and planning. Therefore, this book aims to give our customers everything they need to get all the nutrients that they body needs, especially while doing intense training. In the end, we aim to help our customers live a life that is more focused on having less of an impact on the planet, while maintaining a productive and healthy lifestyle.

BREAKFAST

BANANA CHOCOLATE PANCAKES

Ingredients List:

- 2 bananas, mashed and peeled
- 2 dates or figs, dried with pit removed
- 70g of flour, buckwheat is prefered
- 3-4 tablespoons of linseeds
- 15-20g of amaranth or other ancient grain
- 3-4 tablespoons of plant based protein
- 2-3 tablespoons of chocolate pieces, cacao nibs are preferred
- 200-250ml of non dairy milk, such as hemp milk, almond milk, soy milk, chocolate flavored is preferred
- 200ml of water

Steps:

1. Combine all the ingredients in a large mixing bowl.

2. Pour a small amount of neutral oil such as coconut oil or canola oil onto a large, flat pan. Spread this around, making sure it covers the entire surface area. This is essential to avoid sticking.
3. Preheat the pan on medium heat. Be careful not to overheat the pan, as this would cause the pancakes to scorch when they are poured on. When the oil begins to look shiny, it should be hot enough.
4. Pour small amount of the mixture on the pan until the desired pancake size is reached. Try to keep them small enough to flip easily. Pancakes that are too large become problematic and may not cook consistently.
5. Each pancake should take 3-5 minutes on the first side. However, this may vary depending on the type of pan used, the temperature of the burner, etc. You should check periodically to make sure the pancake is not burning. When it is golden brown, flip to the other side with a spatula.
6. The other side of the pancake should take about two minutes to finish cooking. When golden brown, remove from pan.

Notes: Pancakes are a versatile breakfast food, in that many of the ingredients can be interchanged according to taste. For example, if you don't like bananas, then try blueberries, raspberries, apples, etc. If you don't like dates or figs, try any other fruit that can provide the same level of sweetness. If you can't find ancient grains like amaranth, then feel free to exclude this from the recipe by adding in more flour. You can also try experimenting with different types of flours, as there are many vegan options now in health food stores. Use this recipe as a jumping off point and make it your own!

OATMEAL WITH FRUIT AND NUTS

Ingredients List:

- 2-3 cups of non dairy milk, plain almond milk is preferred
- 1-2 bananas, ripened is preferred
- ½ cup of chopped walnuts
- 2-3 cups of oats, steel cut oats are preferred
- ¼ teaspoon of vanilla extract
- ¼ teaspoon of almond extract
- 2-3 tablespoons of cocoa powder, unsweetened is preferred
- Cinnamon to taste, a pinch is usually enough
- Chocolate chips to taste
- 2-3 tablespoons of agave syrup
- Salt to taste

Steps:

1. Dice the bananas and bring the non dairy milk up to a simmer in a medium size saucepan. Make sure not to burn the milk, as it has a tendency to stick to the bottom of the pan.

2. Combine the diced bananas, the almond extract, the vanilla extract, the agave syrup, and salt in the saucepan. Bring to a boil, while stirring constantly.

3. Put the rest of the ingredients except the chopped walnuts in the pan and reduce the heat to medium. At this point, you should be extra careful that the saucepan does not get too hot, as it may boil over or burn on the bottom. If the saucepan gets too hot remove from heat immediately, let cool, lower the heat, and return to burner.

4. Oats should take about 5-7 minutes to cook. When the oats are soft, transfer to 2-4 bowls depending on the amount desired and the amount of people eating. Before serving, sprinkle the chopped walnuts on top.

Notes: There are a lot of different places this recipe can go, so feel free to use your imagination. For example, if you don't like walnuts, then you can replace these with almonds. If you can't find agave syrup, find another natural source of sweetness, such as honey. If you don't like bananas pretty much any other fruit will do. Different types of berries are usually a good alternative. If you can't find vanilla extract, perhaps trying a non dairy milk that is vanilla flavored. Don't be afraid to experiment!

Breakfast Burrito

Ingredients List:

- 1 16oz package of tofu, firm and unseasoned is preferred
- 6 tortillas, whole grain is preferred
- 1-2 cloves of garlic
- 1 medium sized onion
- ½-1 cup of salsa
- ½ teaspoon of salt
- 1-2 teaspoons of olive oil
- Black pepper to taste, freshly ground is preferred

Steps:

1. Drain the tofu from the water in the packaging and crumble into small pieces into a bowl. Dice onion and garlic. Add as much of each as you would like.
2. Preheat a medium frying pan on medium heat and then add 1-2 teaspoons of olive oil. When olive oil begins to shimmer, add diced onion and garlic to the frying pan. Sprinkle a pinch of salt on the top. You should stir the onions and garlic to avoid burning and to make sure that they cook evenly. These

should cook for about 4-5 minutes, depending on the type of pan used and the temperature.

3. When the onions turn translucent, add the crumbled tofu on top of the onions and garlic. Add in another pinch of salt and as much pepper as you would like. A pinch of two is usually sufficient.

4. This mixture should cook for 3-5 minutes. Make sure to stir periodically. After this time, turn off heat and spoon the desired amount of the mixture into the tortillas. After this, top with as much salsa as you would like.

Notes: This recipe does not offer a whole lot of freedom, at least when compared with previous recipes. You can try using different types of salsa, as there are a wide variety of them. However, if this is a pre-workout meal, try not to get salsas that are too spicy, as this might irritate the digestive tract and interrupt your exercise. You can also try different types of tortillas or even different types of bread to make a sandwich. Just make sure that they are not made with animal fat, as some of the more authentic tortillas are made with pork fat. Perhaps you can even try adding in different seasons, such as tumeric or cumin. Just be careful with these because they can be powerful and overwhelm the dish.

WAFFLES

Ingredients List:

- 2 cups of flour, whole wheat is preferred
- 1-2 bananas, fully ripened is preferred
- ½ cup of soy milk or almond milk
- ½ cup of baking soda
- 1 teaspoon of salt
- 1-2 teaspoons of lemon juice
- 1 cup of applesauce

Steps:

1. Preheat a waffle iron and mash the banana in a medium bowl.
2. Combine the rest of the ingredients in the same bowl as the banana. Mix this vigorously to get rid of the lumps. It might be advisable to mix the wet ingredients and the dry ingredients separately and then combine. However, this is optional.
3. When the waffle iron is up to temperature, spray it liberally with a cooking spray to make it non stick. Then pour in the mixture to cover the waffle molds. However, when the lid is

put down, the batter will squeeze out the sides if you put too much in. Make sure not to put too much batter or this will cause a mess. Each waffle should take about 5 minutes to cook or until golden brown.

4. When the waffle is finished, use a flat spatula or a butter knife to remove it from the mold. Continue to pour more waffles until batter is finished.

Notes: This recipe is very adaptable, as a lot of different ingredients can be interchanged. That is, many people enjoy a wide variety of fruits, which can both be put into the batter or layered on top when served. Waffles can also be served powdered sugar, syrups, jams, jellies, or anything else to make it sweet. Furthermore, typical waffle recipes call for eggs, but, in this case the eggs were replaced with applesauce, which help them achieve the same consistency. However, there are many other replacements for eggs, some of which are commercial products. Each of these gives a slightly different result, so you should experiment with each and decide which works best for you.

LUNCH

LENTIL BOWL

Ingredients List:

- 2 cups of lentils, green ones are preferred
- 2 tablespoons of tomato paste
- 4 tablespoons of olive oil
- 1 large leek, only the white parts
- 2 cloves of garlic
- 4 tablespoons of soy sauce, low sodium variety is preferred
- Salt and pepper to taste
- 5 cups of water

Steps:

1. Preheat a medium frying pan on medium heat. Finely chop garlic and leeks.

2. Add olive oil to pan and let it come up to temperature. When the oil is shimmering, add the garlic, leeks, and tomato paste to the frying pan. Stir continuously to avoid the tomato paste burning, as it has a tendency to stick to the bottom of the frying pan.

3. When fragrant, add the lentils and the water to the frying pan. Bring the mixture up to a boil. Then reduce the heat, cover the pan with a lid, and simmer. Make sure to stir from time to time to ensure everything cooks evenly.

4. When the tomato paste begins to darken and the lentils are tender, remove from heat and let it sit covered for about 10 minutes. Then add the soy sauce, salt, and pepper to your desired taste.

Notes: Lentils are a versatile food that goes well with many different types of ingredients. If you want, you can add a variety of vegetables, such as onion, squash, zucchini, broccoli, bell peppers, among many others. Just add these in when you put in the garlic, leaks, and tomato paste. This dish would also go well with spices that are common in Indian and Middle Eastern cuisines, such as curry powder and turmeric. Be careful, though, to add these cautiously, as they can be powerful.

FLAXSEED BURGER

Ingredients List:

- 3 cloves of garlic
- 1-2 cups of nuts, almonds or walnuts are preferred
- 6-7 tablespoons of flaxseeds
- 2 ½ cups of coconut oil
- 2 ½ cups of apple cider vinegar
- 1 large tomato
- Half of a large red onion
- ¼ of a head of romaine lettuce
- Pickles if desired
- Ketchup or mustard if desired
- Salt and pepper to taste

Steps:

1. Combine all of the ingredients into a blender. Pulse the blender until the ingredients become emulsified. Then, blend until smooth, creating a consistency that can be molded.

2. After this, remove the mixture and create as many patties of whatever size you find acceptable. This is really up to you, as you can many small patties or a few large ones.
3. Heat a medium sized frying pan and place in coconut oil. When oil is melted, place in patties. Be careful to place away from you, as the oil may splatter. Each side should only take 2-3 minutes to cook.
4. When both sides are golden brown, remove from frying pan. Then take two slices per patty of whole wheat bread and place them into the frying pan. Fry both sides until golden brown.
5. Remove slices of bread from frying pan, arrange on a plate, and place patties on them.
6. Slice the large tomato and onion into thin slices and place on top of the patty. Put as many or as little as you desire, depending on your tastes. Rip off 1 or 2 leaves of romaine lettuce, wash thoroughly, and put on top of the patty as well. Apply ketchup or mustard as wish, again, depending on how you like it.

Notes: These types of burgers can any condiments that you like. Some people like adding pickled onions and garlic, some people like adding mayonnaise, others like adding sriracha. A handful of people like adding sliced beets. You can also use a variety of different types of buns, such as those made with potato, to give it a unique taste. Furthermore, if you cannot find or do not like coconut oil, it is possible to use other oils, such as canola oil, sunflower seed oil, olive oil, etc. It is also possible to replace the apple cider vinegar with a juice concentrate or even white vinegar, as long as you aware that white vinegar will have a stronger flavor, so use it sparingly. Also, if you want to add other leaves instead of romaine feel free. Spinach and kale are a great alternative, although be sure to remove the dense kale spine before using.

SEED PIZZA

Ingredients List:

- 250g of sunflower seeds
- 200g of chickpeas
- 70ml of coconut oil
- ½ tablespoon of curry powder
- ½ tablespoon of turmeric
- 1 medium sized sweet potato
- 1 onion, red onion is preferred
- Half of a head of broccoli
- Half of a head of cauliflower

Steps:

1. Preheat the oven to 350 degrees
2. Combine the sunflower seeds, the chickpeas, the coconut oil, the curry powder, and the turmeric. This will create a dough like consistency that will be used to make the base of the pizza. However, it may need to be worked more by hand for it to form the desired consistency.

3. When this is reached, grease a baking tray with coconut oil. Then, place the dough on the tray. Mold the dough into the desired shape, making sure to make its thickness as even as possible. If not, this will cause it to cook at different rates, leaving some parts undercooked, while other are overcooked.
4. After this, slice the sweet potato into thin slices. Then chop the broccoli and cauliflower into bite size pieces. Distributed all of these on top of the dough. Do not put too much in one area, as this may result in the dough being undercooked or becoming soggy.
5. Once the oven is up to the desired temperature, place the baking sheet into the oven. It should take 45 minutes to cook, although this time can be adjusted based on your desire. If you like a softer pizza, consider leaving it in for 40 minutes. If you like a crispier pizza, perhaps leave it in for 50 minutes.
6. When the pizza is to your liking, take out of the oven and let cool before slicing. If you slice while it is still hot, then it will not have enough time to set and become firm. Use a knife or a pizza cutter to cut the pizza into triangles or squares, whichever is most appropriate, and serve.

Notes: The crust for this pizza can be made out of many different types of seeds, although it needs the chickpeas due to their bonding capabilities.

VEGETABLE AND BEAN SOUP

Ingredients List:

- 2 cups of dried beans, any type will do, but kidney beans are preferred
- 2 large onions
- 3 large carrots
- 3 stalks of celery
- 2 bell peppers
- 4 gloves of garlic
- 6 large button mushrooms
- 1 tablespoon of salt
- Fresh cracked pepper to taste
- 2 bay leaves
- 3 tablespoons of olive oil
- 2 teaspoons of tomato paste

Steps:

1. Soak dried beans overnight in lukewarm water. Fill up a large pot with 3 parts water and 1 part beans. This will soften the

beans as they absorb the water. By the time you are ready to cook, you should be able to break them between your fingers.

2. Finely chop all of the onions, carrots, bell pepper, mushrooms, and celery. The size does not matter all that much, as most of it will break down through the cooking process.

3. Once this is done, preheat a large soup pot on medium heat. Add olive oil to the bottom of the pot along with the chopped onions. These need to be sauteed until the onions turn translucent, as this helps intensify the flavor.

4. At this point, add in the chopped celery, carrots, mushrooms, and bell peppers. Sautee these on medium heat for 10 to 15 minutes. Be sure to stir periodically and to scrape the bottom of the pot if anything starts to stick. A lot of moisture will be released in this stage, significantly reducing the size of the chopped vegetables.

5. After this, finely chop the cloves of garlic and add to the pot. Make sure to stir so that the garlic does not burn.

6. When all of the vegetables are almost finished, add in the tomato paste, salt, and crack as much pepper as you would like. This should be cooked until the tomato paste begins to change to a darker color.

7. After this, drain the beans of the excess water that they have been soaking in and add them to the pot. Also add in about 2 liters of fresh water and the bay leaves. This should simmer for about 30 minutes. During this time, stir and make sure the bottom of the pot is free from any sticking material.

8. When finished, serve in a large soup bowl. You can add extra salt and pepper according to your preference at this stage.

Notes: Many different types of beans can be used in this soup, including navy beans, lima beans, black beans, etc. However, you should know that the larger the bean the more time it takes to soak, so adjust your soak times accordingly. Furthermore, this soup can accommodate a lot of different types of vegetables, so feel free to add in whatever you like. That is, the base of the soup is made up of carrots, bell peppers, onions, garlic, and celery, but spinach, kale, squash, etc. can be added as well. These do not need to saute and can be added in half way through step 7 to give them adequate time to soften up and become edible.

PEPPERS STUFFED WITH QUINOA

- 4-5 poblano or bell peppers
- 2-3 teaspoons of olive oil
- 1 cup of red quinoa
- 1 cup of vegetable broth, low sodium is preferred
- 2 garlic cloves
- 1 large onion
- 3/4 cup of corn, cooked or thawed
- 1 cup of previous soaked black beans
- 1 teaspoon of chili powder
- 1 small can of diced green chiles, mild is preferred
- 1/2 teaspoon of cumin
- Salt and freshly ground black pepper to taste
- 3 tablespoons of vegan cheese
- Cilantro, freshly chopped if desired
- Greek yogurt, non flavored

Steps:

1. Preheat the broiler on your oven to medium high, but move the oven rack down to second position, as the food will burn if they are too close to the heat source.

2. Take the poblano peppers and rub them liberally with olive oil. After this, put them into a non stick pan that is safe for the oven. If you have a cast iron skillet that is well seasoned, then this would be good in this situation. Put the peppers into the oven for 5 minutes or until you see the skin of the peppers start to blister. Flip the peppers and repeat this process.

3. After this, take the peppers out of the oven. Put them in a large bowl and cover them with plastic wrap. Let them sit for about 10 minutes, which gives them time to steam from their own heat and moisture. At this point, move the oven rack to the middle of the oven and set the oven to 350 degrees, but do not put the peppers back into the oven yet.

4. While waiting for the peppers to rest in the bowl, put the quinoa in a strainer and run cold water over them for 1-2 minutes to clean them properly. After this, bring a medium sized pot up to temperature on medium heat, and then add 1 teaspoon of olive oil to the bottom. Once the oil is hot, put the quinoa in and stir for about 1 minute. This will toast the quinoa, imparting a rich and deep flavor.

5. At this point, add in the vegetable broth and 3/4 cup of water. Bring this mixture up to a boil, and then cover with a lid. Reduce the heat to low and allow it to simmer for about 15 minutes. When the quinoa is cooked, take it off the heat and let it sit without the lid for 5 more minutes.

6. While this is happening, preheat a small frying pan and add in 1 teaspoon of olive oil. Bring the oil up to temperature and then add in the diced onions and garlic. Stir this continuously, as the garlic may burn. Cook this for about 5-7 minutes. If the garlic and onions begin to brown, then take them off the heat.

7. After this, put the cooked onions and garlic in a large bowl, along with the quinoa, beans, green chiles, chili powder, corn, cumin, salt, and pepper. Mix this so that the ingredients are evenly distributed.

8. Take the peppers out of the bowl and peel off the skin. These should come off easily. If they do not, do not worry. Take as much off as you can. Cut the peppers in half long ways and remove the seeds. Put the peppers back into the same pan that

you broiled them in and begin to fill them with the mixture from the large bowl. When finished, put as much of the vegan cheese on top as you would like. However, do not put too much, as it may melt on to the bottom of the pan and burn while in the oven.

9. Lastly, put the peppers back in the oven and bake them for about 15 minutes or until they are heated all the way through. When finished, remove from the oven, put more cheese on top if desired and top with the chopped cilantro and greek yoghurt.

Notes: This dish can also be done with any peppers you like, although poblanos tend to have the best tasted, especially when roasted. If you can't find poblanos try using green, red, or yellow bell peppers. You can also try adding in different vegetables to the stuffing mixture, such as squash, spinach, kale, etc. However, be sure to chop these vegetable additions small to ensure that they cook properly.

CHICKPEA SANDWICH WITH ROASTED SUNFLOWER SEEDS

Ingredients List:

- 1 large can of chickpeas, drained and rinsed
- 1/3 cup of sunflower seeds, roasted and unsalted is preferred
- 1/2 tsp of mustard, spicy mustard or dijon mustard is preferred
- 3 tablespoons of vegan mayo
- 1/2 of a large red onion
- 1 tablespoon of maple syrup
- 2-3 tablespoons of dill
- Salt and pepper to taste
- 4 pieces of whole wheat bread bread
- 1 avocado
- 1 large tomato
- ¼ head of romaine lettuce
- 1/4 cup of hummus, unflavored is preferred
- 1/2 of a medium sized lemon
- 2 cloves of garlic
- 1 cup of almond milk, unsweetened is preferred

Steps:

1. To make the garlic sauce, first finely chop the garlic and put into a small bowl. Then, squeeze the half lemon and add the humus into the same bowl. Stir this mixture until the ingredients are evenly distributed. After this, pour the almond milk in slowly until the desired consistency is achieved. For those who like thick sauce, add in less. For those who want it more runny, add in more almond milk. Set this garlic aside until later.

2. Add the chickpeas to a large bowl and mash them with whisk, fork, or any other tool that works well. After this, add the roasted sunflower seeds and mash as well. If the sunflower seeds are not roasted, then put them in a dry pan on low heat until they begin to change color. Once everything is mashed, put in the vegan mayo, the mustard, the diced red onion, the maple syrup, and the dill. Mix this together and add the salt and pepper to your desired flavor.

3. After this, take the bread and toast them if this is how you like it. Take one or more scoops of the mixture and apply to the center of the bread. Press down gently so that the mixture is even on the bread. At this point, put as much or as little of the garlic sauce as you would like.

Notes: This recipe has numerous places for substitution if you cannot find or do not like one or more of the ingredients. For example, instead of chickpeas, you can try pretty much any other type of beans. Just make sure that they are soft enough to mash, especially if you are starting from dried beans. Perhaps try black beans, kidney beans, lima beans, or navy beans. Each has a different flavor so be sure to experiment and find what works for you. You can also try different types of sweetner instead of the maple syrup. For example, you can try agave nectar or juice concentrates. Again, just be sure to add them sparingly and taste as you go, as you cannot remove them once added. Furthermore, this recipe would be good with many different types of herbs in addition to the dill. That is, parsely, basil, and cilantro would work with the other ingredients. Feel free to chop them finely and add them to the mixture.

ROASTED PUMPKIN SOUP

Ingredients List:

- One medium size pumpkin or 4 large cans of pumpkin
- Salt and pepper to taste
- ½ teaspoon of nutmeg
- 4 cups of vegetable stock
- One large yellow onion
- 3 gloves of garlic
- 4 cups of coconut milk
- 2 teaspoons of maple syrup
- 4 tablespoons of olive oil
- 1 loaf of french bread

Steps:

1. If you are starting with an actual pumpkin, cut it in half and remove the seeds and the soft parts of the inside. Save as many of the seeds as possible and discard the pumpkin guts. From here, remove the outer layer of the pumpkin and

discard. Cut the remaining pumpkin parts into 1 inch chunks and place them in a large mixing bowl.

2. Preheat the oven to 350 degrees. Add in 2 tablespoons of olive oil, along with a large pinch of salt and a large pinch of freshly cracked pepper. Mixed this thoroughly and then dump the contents of the bowl onto a large cookie sheet, making sure to spread the pumpkin chunks evenly. Place the cookie sheet in the oven and bake for 15-20 minutes. Flip the pumpkin chunks over and bake for another 10-15 minutes. This should give them a golden brown color, which will impart a lot of flavor to the soup.

3. While the pumpkin is in the oven, preheat a large soup pot on the stove. Dice the entire onion. This may seem like a lot of onions, but it will break down and virtually disappear. Add in the remaining olive oil to the pot and bring this up to temperature. When the olive oil is shimmering, add in the onion and another pinch of salt and pepper. Saute this until the onions become translucent. At this point, dice the garlic and add this into the mixture. Saute this for about 2 minutes, making sure to stir so that the garlic does not burn.

4. When the pumpkin is finished, remove it from the oven and add it to the large soup pot. Also, add in the vegetable stock and bring up to a boil. Once boiling, lower the heat and let it simmer for about 10 minutes.

5. While the soup is simmering, cut the french bread into half inch slices, season with olive oil, salt, and pepper. Place these on a large baking sheet and put in the oven. These should take 3 minutes to toast, but every oven is different, so check this regularly to avoid burning them.

6. At this point, add in the coconut milk and stir. If you have a handheld blender, use this to blend the soup until it is a smooth consistency. If you do not have a handheld blender, then add to a blender with a large ladle. Be careful transferring the soup and operating the blender because you will get burned.

7. Once the soup has been blended, you are ready to serve. Ladle the soup into medium sized soup bowls, sprinkle with

nutmeg, and top with a piece or two of the toasted bread. You can add in the maple syrup to give it a sweeter flavor, but this step is optional and should be done to your preferences.

Notes: Soups like this are very adaptable, in that many other types of ingredients can be added. For example, try baking carrots alongside the pumpkin and adding them to the soup. This will give the soup a sweeter and slightly Earthy flavor. You can also try adding sweet potatoes in the same way. This will help the soup thicken up and give a richer flavor. In general, the pumpkin is the base of the soup, but you can anywhere you like after that. Try other vegetables and roast and blend them in with the pumpkin to create a unique flavor. You can also try adding in different herbs. Parsely, basil, and rosemary would work well here. Just add them in slowly and taste as you go, as you cannot take them out once you put them in.

Broccoli, Asparagus, Carrot, and Pea Soup

Ingredients List:

- 2 large heads of broccoli
- 10 stalks of asparagus
- 4 cups of peas, fresh or frozen is fine
- 1 large yellow onion
- 2 large carrots
- 3 cloves of garlic
- 3 tablespoons of olive oil
- Salt and pepper to taste
- 4 cups of vegetable stock
- 1 loaf of french bread
- ½ tablespoon of paprika

Steps:

1. Begin by finely chopping the onion and preheating a large soup pot on the stove. Add in all of the olive oil and bring it up to temperature. Once it begins to simmer, add in the onion

and saute, stirring periodically. While this is happening, dice all of the garlic. Once the onions begin to brown, which should take 10-15 minutes, add in the garlic. Saute this for about 2 minutes, allowing the garlic to release its oils.

2. At this point, add in the vegetable stock and let the mixture simmer on the stove while you prepare the other ingredients. Wash and chop the broccoli, asparagus, and carrots. Make sure to remove tough parts, such as the stem of the broccoli and the base of the asparagus stalks. Chop these into small chunks and put into the soup pot, along with the peas.

3. Cover the soup mixture, bring it up to a boil, and then lower the heat and let it simmer for 20 minutes. At this point, the vegetables should be soft, so blend the mixture with a handheld blender. If you do not have one, transfer the mixture to a blender with a ladle. Of course, be careful here, as the soup is extremely hot and the blender can shoot the liquid upwards. Blend this until smooth.

4. After this, take the french bread and slice it into half inch slices. Drizzle olive oil on these and season with salt and pepper. Cook these in a toaster oven or regular oven until they are golden brown.

5. At this point, you are ready to serve. Ladle the soup into medium sized soup bowls and top with as many pieces of the toasted french bread as you would like. Also, sprinkle some fresh cracked pepper and salt on top of the soup to taste. If desired, drizzle olive oil on top as well.

Notes: This recipe can be changed as you desire, as this is just one example of how to make a delicious vegetable soup. That is, each of the vegetables can be switched out with pretty much anything else you like, although this combination tends to work well together. You can also add potatoes to this, which will create a thicker and starchier soup. Perhaps try adding in kale or spinach, although be sure to remove the spine of the kale leaves, as these can be bitter and tough to eat. This soup is also a good base to which you can add beans or tofu if you want to get more protein. Just cook these separately and add them to the soup after it has been blended.

Spinach, Red Cabbage, and Herb Salad

Ingredients List:

- 8 cups of loose spinach leaves
- ¼ of a large red cabbage
- ½ cup of fresh basil
- ½ cup of fresh mint
- ½ cup of fresh cilantro
- ½ cup of fresh parsley
- ½ cup of aged balsamic vinegar
- ½ cup of extra virgin olive oil
- ½ cup of dijon or whole grain mustard
- Salt and pepper to taste

Steps:

1. Take the red cabbage and cut it into 1/4ths. Cut off the white and tough stem, as it is inedible. Chop the red cabbage into bite sized pieces and then place these into a large salad bowl. Add in the spinach as well.

2. Take the herbs and lightly chop these as well. Make sure to remove any tough stems. Smaller and softer stems are fine to include, although try to limit the amount of them. When finished, put these herbs into the bowl.
3. Take a large jar with a lid that secures tightly, such as mason jar. In this jar, pour in the balsamic vinegar, the olive oil, and the mustard. Add in a pinch of salt and freshly cracked pepper if you desire. Shake this vigorously until it emulsifies. It should look like a smooth sauce, without any noticeable separation of the individual components. At this point, taste the dressing to add more of each ingredient to make it your own.
4. Mix the salad well and serve in a medium sized salad bowl. Add the dressing over the salad, as much or as little as you like.

Notes: Like most salads, many different types of ingredients can be added. For example, you can add beets, broccoli, cucumbers, squash, among many others. You can also remove as many of the herbs as you like, if you cannot find them or if you do not like them. Furthermore, be sure to use high quality olive oil and balsamic vinegar in this case. Because these ingredients are not being cooked, you will be able to taste them far more, meaning low quality ingredients have the potential to ruin the dressing. Likewise, try to find high quality mustard, and do not use yellow mustard for this. If you can't find high quality ingredients for the dressing, consider using a commercial brand dressing, as there are many vegan options.

VINAIGRETTE PASTA SALAD

Ingredients List:

- 2 cups of small cut pasta, any will do
- Half of a head of broccoli
- 1 zucchini
- ¼ of a red cabbage
- Half of a red onion
- ½ cup of aged balsamic vinegar
- ½ cup of extra virgin olive oil
- Half cup or mustard, dijon or whole grain mustard is preferred
- 1 cup of vegan cheese
- ½ cup of pine nuts

Steps:

1. Chop the all of the vegetables to bite sized pieces. Be sure to remove inedible parts, such as the core of the red cabbage and the stem of the broccoli. Combine all of these into a large salad bowl, along with the pine nuts.

2. Bring a large pot of water up to a boil and add in the pasta. Any type of small pasta will do, as long as it is roughly bite sized. Avoid long pasta strands. Once the pasta is soft, pour the pasta and the water into a strainer. The past should take 5-7 minutes to cook.

3. While leaving the pasta to continue draining in the sink to remove any remaining water, mix the dressing in a jar with a lid that closes securely, such as a mason jar. In this jar, pour in the balsamic vinegar, the olive oil, and the mustard. Shake vigorously until the entire mixture is emulsified, without any noticeable separation.

4. After this, you are ready to serve. Pour the pasta into the salad bowl and mix to evenly distribute all of the ingredients. Serve into a medium sized salad bowl and drizzle as much dressing over the top as you would like. Add in the vegan cheese on the top.

Notes: Feel free to experiment with different types of pastas, but, of course, only use the ones that do not contain eggs. That is, some types of pasta are made with just flour and water, while others contain eggs, so be careful to read the ingredients list before buying. Also, you can add in a wide variety of other vegetables to this recipe. For example, try adding in different types of leaves, like chinese cabbage, arugula, spinach, kale, etc. Also, the pine nuts can be substituted for other types in case you are allergic or simply do not like them. Try adding in walnuts or almonds. For an extra twist, you can toast the nuts before adding them in by putting them in a frying pan and slowly heating them without oil until they are golden brown.

RED DAL

Ingredients List:

- 2 cups of red lentils
- 1 large onion, yellow or red is fine
- 1 large tomato, canned is fine by fresh is preferred
- ½ teaspoon of cayenne pepper
- 1 teaspoon of cumin
- ½ teaspoon of turmeric
- 1 teaspoon of coriander
- Salt and pepper to taste
- 2 teaspoons of cumin seeds
- 2 tablespoons of olive or vegetable oil
- 1 teaspoon of mustard seeds, black or yellow seeds are fine
- 1 cup of curry leaves, frozen is fine but fresh is preferred
- 14 ounces of coconut milk

Steps:

1. Chop the onion and tomato finely and add it to a large saucepan. Then add the lentils, cayenne pepper, cumin,

coriander, and salt and pepper to taste. Cover the ingredients with water and bring to a boil. Cook this for about 30 minutes, which is about enough time for the lentils to start to break down.

2. At this point, preheat a medium sized frying pan and add the vegetable oil over medium heat. Once the oil is shimmering, put in the cumin and the mustard seeds. Have a lid ready to cover this pan, as the seeds will start to pop. This should not take long before this begins. When this happens reduce the heat until the popping stops and then add the onion, which has been finely chopped, and the curry leaves. Cook all of these together for 2-3 minutes or until golden brown. The leaves will burn if left unattended, so make sure to stir regularly.

3. Add the contents of the frying pan to the large saucepan. Stir this together. At this point, the contents should be a somewhat smooth soft paste. Add in salt and pepper to your liking, and sprinkle in the chopped curry leaves if you desire. Also, at this time you should add in the coconut milk. Put in as little or as much as you desire, but usually a small splash per dish is enough. Serve in a small dish.

Notes: This dish goes well with naan or garlic bread. Naan is a traditional bread from Indian and the Middle East, also where this dish originates. You can buy naan at most stores, and it can easily by heating it in the oven until warm. Also, the curry leaves may be difficult to find, as they are a specialty item. If you cannot find them, it is fine to leave them out or replace them with a small sprinkle of curry powder. You might want to also try adding in spinach to this recipe. Simply chop it and add it into the saucepan with the lentils. Spinach will shrink considerably and mix smoothly with the rest of the mixture.

DINNER:

BLACK BEAN BAKED POTATO

Ingredients List:

- 2 large russet potatoes
- 2 cups of dried black beans
- ½ of a large onion, red is fine by white is preferred
- ½ cup of fresh cilantro
- 1 large jalapeno pepper
- 2 tablespoons of coconut oil
- Salt and pepper to taste
- 2 cups of vegan cheese
- Hot sauce, such as Tabasco
- 1 large bell pepper
- 4 cups of vegetable stock

Steps:

1. The night before, soak the black beans in a large pot with twice as much water as the beans. By the time you are ready to cook, these should be soft enough to easily bite through. Drain the water and replace with vegetable stock. Boil this until the beans are soft and the liquid has reduced by half.
2. At this point, take the two potatoes and stab numerous holes into them with a fork. This allows them to cook evenly. Place them in an oven safe baking dish, preheat the oven to 400 degrees, and place them in the oven for 30 minutes. Before taking them out, check to see if you easily pierce them to the center with a knife. If not, leave in the oven until you can do this.
3. Put the potatoes on a plate and cut them in half lengthwise. Salt and pepper the inside of the potatoes with as little or as much as you would like. Liberally apply the coconut to both potatoes. Sprinkle the vegan cheese on the hot surface of the potatoes that it can begin to melt. Chop the onion, bell pepper, and the cilantro finely and sprinkle over the top as well. If you desire, chop the jalapeno and put on as much as you would like. Likewise, use as much of the hot sauce as you wish. Lastly, scoop the black beans on top.

Notes: This recipe can also be done with sweet potatoes, although the white russet potato is the classic way to do it. Sweet potatoes has a very different flavor, as they impart a lot more sweetness, so use these cautiously. You can also incorporate many other types of herbs, such as basil and parsley. However, this is largely inspired by Mexican flavors, so use these sparingly, as they may conflict with the other flavors. Also, if you are going to use the jalapeno, make sure to remove the seeds and the inner white parts, as these contain most of the spiciness, unless you can tolerate this level of spice. Furthermore, you can try using other types of beans, such as kidney beans, although black beans fit better with the Mexican inspired flavors. Pinto beans might be a good alternative.

VEGETABLE PASTA

Ingredients List:

- 4 large cans of crushed tomatoes
- 1 large onion
- 4 cloves of garlic
- 1 large head of broccoli
- 1 large head of cauliflower
- 1 medium sized box of spaghetti
- 4 tablespoons of olive oil
- Salt and pepper to taste
- 2 cups of red wine
- 2 bay leaves
- 1 teaspoon of oregano
- 1 cup of fresh basil

Steps:

1. To make the spaghetti sauce, begin be chopping the large onion as finely as possible. Then, preheat a large soup pot and add the olive oil to the bottom. Bring the olive oil up to

temperature and when it begins to shimmer add in the chopped onion. Cook the onion for about 15 minutes, stirring continuously. While this may seem like a long time, onions contain a lot of water which needs to be removed to allow for them to slightly brown.

2. When the onions begin to take on a bit of color, chop the cloves of garlic and add them to the pot. Continue to cook and stir the garlic and onion for another 2-3 minutes. Then add in the red wine. Cook this until it reduces by half to allow for the alcohol to burn off, thus intensifying the flavor.

3. At this point, add in the 4 cans of tomatoes and stir the mixture together. Take one of the empty cans, fill it with water, and add it to the pot. This helps it avoid becoming too thick and sticking to the bottom of the pot. Now, add in the oregano, the bay leaves, and salt and pepper to your liking. Bring this mixture up to a biol, cover with a lid, and then reduce the heat. Let the sauce simmer for at least 30 minutes, although the more it simmers the better the flavor. Stir the pot every few minutes, making sure to scrap the bottom, as the sauce may stick and burn.

4. When the sauce is finished, bring a large pot of water up to a boil and add in the pasta. At this same time, chop the broccoli and the cauliflower into bite sized pieces, making sure to remove all of the inedible pieces such as the stem. Put this into the sauce as it simmers, thus allowing the vegetables to soften, which should happen in 5 to 10 minutes.

5. The past should take about 8 minutes to cook. When it is finished, drain the water and the pasta into a strainer. Serve in a large bowl by putting the pasta on the bottom and spooning as much sauce and vegetables as you would like over the top. Before serving chop and sprinkle the leaves of basil over the top, again using as much as you would like.

Notes: Of course, you can add it pretty much any vegetables that you like to the sauce. For example, you can try adding carrots, squash, zucchini, or even cabbage. However, you should be aware that different vegetables take different amounts of time to cook, depending on how dense they are. Therefore, allow more time for vegetables like carrots to cook in the sauce. This recipe also works well with any type of pasta that you can find, as long as it does not contain eggs. If you can find pasta or if you would prefer something else, try serving this over a bed of rice. The sauce could also be served with a few pieces of toast if rice is not your thing either. This is a versatile sauce that can be applied pretty much anywhere. Experiment and find out which is best for you.

VEGAN LASAGNA

Ingredients List:

- 4 large cans of crushed tomatoes
- 1 large onion, white or yellow is preferred
- 4 cloves of garlic
- 4 tablespoons of olive oil
- Salt and pepper to taste
- 2 cups of red wine
- 2 bay leaves
- 1 teaspoon of oregano
- 1 cup of fresh basil
- 4 cups of vegan cheese
- 1 box of large lasagna noodles
- 3 large portobello mushrooms

Steps:

1. To make the spaghetti sauce, begin be chopping the large onion as finely as possible. Then, preheat a large soup pot and add the olive oil to the bottom. Bring the olive oil up to

temperature and when it begins to shimmer add in the chopped onion. Cook the onion for about 15 minutes, stirring continuously. While this may seem like a long time, onions contain a lot of water which needs to be removed to allow for them to slightly brown.

2. When the onions begin to take on a bit of color, chop the cloves of garlic and add them to the pot. Continue to cook and stir the garlic and onion for another 2-3 minutes. Then add in the red wine. Cook this until it reduces by half to allow for the alcohol to burn off, thus intensifying the flavor.

3. At this point, add in the 4 cans of tomatoes and stir the mixture together. Take one of the empty cans, fill it with water, and add it to the pot. This helps it avoid becoming too thick and sticking to the bottom of the pot. Now, add in the oregano, the bay leaves, and salt and pepper to your liking. Bring this mixture up to a biol, cover with a lid, and then reduce the heat. Let the sauce simmer for at least 30 minutes, although the more it simmers the better the flavor. Stir the pot every few minutes, making sure to scrap the bottom, as the sauce may stick and burn.

4. When the sauce is finished, take a large baking pan and cover the bottom with a thin layer of the sauce. Put down the first layer of the lasagna noodles. These should still be uncooked at this point, as they will cook in the oven. Otherwise, if you cook them first, they will overcook and become soggy.

5. After this, chop the portobello mushrooms into about 1 centimeter thick slices. Put enough of these on top of the first layer of noodles to create the next layer. The next layer consists of the vegan cheese. Apply this liberally, although reserving enough for future layers. Next, apply a thin layer of sauce to the top.

6. Continue to layer the baking pan, alternating between the layers appropriately. In the end, you should have numerous layers of sauce, uncooked noodles, mushrooms, and vegan cheese.

7. Preheat the oven to 350 degrees. Cover the baking pan with aluminum foil and place in the oven. Let it cook for 30

minutes. At this point, take the aluminum foil off and sprinkle more of the vegan cheese on top. This will allow the top to form a crunchy top. Leave the lasagna in the oven for another 15 minutes.

8. When finished, cut into square pieces and serve. You can add extra sauce if desired. Chop and sprinkle the fresh basil over the top.

Notes: Along with the portobello mushrooms, various other vegetables can be added in as well. For example, spinach works well in this situation, as does kale, assuming the touch spine is removed first. You can also use different types of mushrooms if portobellos are not to your liking or if you do not want to pay the extra cost for them. Also, many stores now cook lasagna noodles that do not need baking, as they can be placed in the lasagna and cooked with other ingredients. This produces better results than traditional methods, as first cooking the noodles and then cooking them in with the other ingredients often leaves them soggy. This meant that the lasagna struggles to hold its shape and the texture lacks any real body, so to avoid this go with the nonboil option.

STIR FRIED NOODLES

Ingredients List:

- 2 large portobello mushrooms, or a dozen small button mushrooms
- ½ of a large white onion
- 2 cloves of garlic
- ½ head of broccoli
- Egg noodles
- Salt and pepper to taste
- ¼ cup of soy sauce
- ¼ cup of teriyaki sauce
- 1 teaspoon of sesame oil

Steps:

1. Chop the onions and garlic finely and place to the side. Chop the mushrooms into thin slices. Chops the broccoli into the size of small bites. Make sure not to leave any thick stems, as these would need much longer to cook.

2. Preheat a medium sized frying pan and add in the sesame oil. When this oil comes up to temperature and begins to shimmer add in the onions and a pinch of salt and pepper. Cook these for about 10 minutes or until they turn translucent. At this point, put in the chopped garlic and cook for another 2 minutes, stirring from time to time to avoid the garlic burning on the bottom of the pan. When finished remove from the heat.

3. While cooking the onions bring a medium size soup pot full of water to a boil. Then, put in the broccoli to blanch it. Let this cook for 1-2 minutes, as you want to maintain some crunch. At this point drain the water and leave to rest on the size. However, save some of the water in a separate pot for use with the noodles.

4. Egg noodles often come dried and only need to be rehydrated, not boiled and cooked like other noodles. Therefore, take the water left over from blanching the broccoli and put the egg noodles in the same pot. Let them soak for 10 minutes.

5. At this point, add the broccoli and the mushrooms to the same frying pan as the garlic and onions and returned to the pan to the heat. Let this cook for 2-3 minutes and then add in the soy sauce and teriyaki sauce. Stir this mixture continuously, as the sauces will thicken and burn. Continue cooking this for another 5-7 minutes.

6. At this point, you are ready to serve. Drain the noodles of their water and place a bed of them at the bottom of a medium sized bowl. Spoon over the broccoli, mushroom, and onions on top of the noodles. If desired, use more soy sauce, teriyaki sauce, or sesame oil to drizzle on top.

Notes: A variety of different types of noodles can be used here, although egg noodles are the traditional choice. If you use different types of noodles, then these most likely need to be cooked by boiling. This dish can also include various amounts of vegetables that you may enjoy. Try different types of mushrooms, especially those that are more common in Asian style cuisines. You can add other vegetables such as cauliflower, squash, chinese cabbage, water chestnuts etc. Just keep in mind that the soy sauce, the teriyaki sauce, and the sesame oil impart very specific and powerful flavors, so try to use extra ingredients that will not conflict with these. When in doubt, try to use ingredients that you have already seen in Chinese, Thai, Japanese, etc. styles. Although this is not a perfect guide, it will help your decision making. However, it is up to you to experiment and find what is best for you.

SNACKS:

RED PEPPER HUMMUS

Ingredients List:

- 4 cups of dried chickpeas
- 4 cloves of garlic
- 3 tablespoons of lemon juice
- 1 tablespoon of salt
- 2 tablespoons of olive oil
- 1 cup of tahini
- 1 red bell pepper
- 6 slices of pita bread

Steps:

1. Begin the process by soaking the dried chickpeas overnight to soften them up. When you are ready to begin cooking, these

should be soft enough to bite through or crush with your fingers.

2. Combine all of the ingredients into a blender and pulse until the mixture is smooth. Taste the mixture and add in more salt, lemon juice, chickpeas, olive oil, garlic, or tahini as needed.
3. Cut the pita bread into triangles and place on a small, oven safe baking sheet. Set the oven to 200 degrees, put the baking sheet in the oven, and let these warm form about 10 minutes.
4. While this is happening, dice the red pepper and mix into the hummus. However, do not blend it in, as you want them to remain as small chunks.
5. Serve into a small bowl, with the warm pita along the outside.

Notes: hummus is a wildly popular dish, as it is served throughout the world. Therefore, you can find a wide variety of different types, such as spinach hummus, beet hummus, garlic hummus, kale hummus, pomegranate hummus, among many others. You can add any of these ingredients into the blender, although some of them need to be prepared before hand. That is, the beets need to either be boiled or baked for 30 minutes to make them soft enough to eat and to blend. You can also feel free to add in various seasonings, such as those that are commonly found in Indian and Middle Eastern cuisine. For example, try adding in curry powder, turmeric, cumin, coriander, paprika, smoked paprika, etc. Like always, add these in a little bit at a time, tasting and adjusting as you go. Remember, once you add these to the mixture, you cannot take them out, so be careful. Hummus can also be added to a wide variety of things as a condiment. For example, when making a sandwich, hummus can spread on each slice, giving the sandwich added texture and flavor.

ANTIOXIDANT SMOOTHIE

Ingredients List:

- 1 cup of frozen berries, any will do but blueberries are preferred
- 1 cup of spinach, kale can be used as well
- ½ cup of frozen banana slices
- 1 tablespoon of flaxseeds
- 1 cup of orange juice
- 1 cup of soy milk

Steps:

1. The night before you should slice your bananas, seal them in a container, and put them in the freezer. This step is important to give your smoothie the texture you are looking for. If you cannot do this, you can add in a cup of ice with the unfrozen banana slices.
2. Take all of the ingredients and put them in a blender. Pulse the blender until the mixture is smooth.

3. Serve the mixture in one or more glasses, depending on how many people are being served. This should be enough for up to 4 people.

Notes: Of course, you can add in as many or as few types of fruit as you would like. Feel free to experiment with pineapple, apples, different types of berries, etc. Most fruits will taste good in the recipe, as long as you enjoy eating the fruit on its own. Also, if you choose to kale, be aware that raw kale can be rather strong tasting. Therefore, be sure to add only a little bit at first and taste the mixture as you add more. Too much kale may make this undrinkable. Also, when using kale be sure to take out the spine, as this is too tough to eat and it may jam up your blender. You can also try using different types of milk and juices, such as almond milk, rice milk, grapefruit juice, apple juice, etc. However, all of these may not go together well so try them first before adding them. For example, grapefruit juice is stronger than most juices and it could conflict with other flavor profiles.

AVOCADO SMOOTHIE

Ingredients List:

- 2 large avocados
- 2 cups of pineapples
- 1 cup of blueberries
- ½ teaspoon of ginger
- 1 cup of vanilla soy milk
- 1 cup of ice

Steps:

1. Take the two avocados and with a sharp knife cut around the seed lengthwise. When you cut into the avocado, keep pressing the knife gently downward until you come to the seed, which is rather large. Rotate the knife around the seed until you come back to where you started, cutting the flesh of the avocado in half. The two halves should separate away from the seed. If this does not happen the avocado might not be ripe enough.
2. While holding one half in your hand, scoop out the flesh of the avocado with a spoon and put into the blender. Also, put

in the rest of the ingredients into the blender and pulse until the mixture is smooth. You can add more ice and blend again to achieve any desired consistency.
3. Pour into glasses to serve. This recipe can serve up to four people comfortably.

Notes: The key ingredient in this recipe is the avocado, yet it is the most difficult to get right. When selecting an avocado from the grocery store it is important to get one that is at the correct level of ripeness. If it is under ripened, then it will be too hard to eat or even blend. If it is overripe, then the flavor might be off or it may be unsafe to eat. Therefore, choose ones that are a little tender to the touch, in that they allow you to push into the skin with a moderate amount of resistance. Don't worry if you cannot find the right ones, as selecting them just takes practice. When it comes to the other fruits, you can use frozen or fresh. However, if you use frozen ones you can reduce the amount of ice that you put into the smoothie. Also, you can experiment with different types of fruits as well, although fruit with a higher citric acid content, such as pineapple, help to balance the rich taste of the avocado. It might also be a good idea to add in a scoop of vegan vanilla ice cream for extra sweetness. This would help it become creamier as well.

SWEET POTATO FRIES

Ingredients List:

- 2 large sweet potatoes
- Salt and pepper to taste
- ¼ cup of olive oil
- 1 tablespoon of garlic powder
- 1 tablespoon of onion powder
- ¼ cup of dried dill
- 1 teaspoon of cayenne pepper

Steps:

1. Preheat the oven to 350 degrees. Then, cut the sweet potatoes into the typical french fried shape. This can be done by first cutting the sweet potatoes in half lengthwise, then cutting them in half again lengthwise. Continue doing this process until you reach a small enough surface area that a french fried shape can be sliced off.
2. After this, put all of the sweet potato piece in a large bowl. Combine them with the rest of the ingredients and stir until everything is evenly coated. Place the sweet potatoes on a

cookie sheet and slide into the oven. These should cook for around 20 minutes in total. However, half way through they need to be flipped. You should also consider rotating the cookie sheet to ensure that everything is cooking evenly.

3. After 20 minutes, the sweet potatoes should be cooked through. At this point, take them out and let them rest for 10 minutes. Turn on the broiler and put the sweet potatoes in the oven again. The broiler is extremely hot and will burn the sweet potatoes if you are not careful. Leave them in for 1 minute, and then take them out, flip them, and return them for another minute. This step is essential to make them crispy on the outside.

Notes: Of course, this recipe can be done with any type of potato, although sweet potatoes have the most nutrition content. You can also try experimenting with different seasonings, such as cumin, curry powders, etc. However, be careful how much you put on the sweet potatoes, as excessive amounts of power will burn, thus totally ruining the snack. You can also try different herbs, although this works well with dill. Perhaps try sage or parsley, as these would certainly give a unique twist. Lastly, just a note of caution, many dishes have been lost due to the broiler, as people underestimate how quickly it will cook food. A few seconds too long and it will burn the dish you just worked so hard to prepare. When it comes to sauces, sweet potato fries work well with the classics like ketchup and mustard, but it may also be a good idea to add in a bit of spice and sweetness with something like sriracha. It is up to you what you want to dip these in, although sweet potatoes do not go well with everything that a normal potato might.

DESSERTS

VEGAN BANANA CREAM PIE

Ingredients List:

- ¾ cup of oats, rolled oats are preferred
- ¾ cup of almonds
- ½ teaspoon of sea salt
- 2 tbsp organic cane sugar or coconut sugar
- ¼ cup coconut oil
- 2 tablespoons of cornstarch
- ⅓ cup of cane sugar
- 1 ½ cups of almond milk, unsweetened is preferred
- 1 teaspoon of vanilla extract
- 1 banana
- 1 14 ounce can of coconut cream
- ½ teaspoon of vanilla extract
- 5 tablespoons of powdered sugar

Steps:

1. Preheat the oven to 350 degrees. Take a medium baking dish and line it with parchment paper. If you don't have parchment paper, you can use coconut oil to grease the pan.

2. In your blender, add in the almonds, the oats, a pinch of salt and the sugar. Pulse the blender until everything is broken down and fully mixed. After this, add in the coconut oil, although make sure it is brought up to room temperature first or this will clump. Pulse the blender again, which will form a dough like consistency. Make sure to scrape the sides during this process, while the blender is not running. If the mixture is too dry add in more coconut oil. In the end, the dough should be pliable and should not crumble to the touch.

3. After this, transfer the dough to the baking dish and spread the dough across the entire surface. Make sure that the thickness is as even as you can get it to ensure that everything cooks evenly. Once this is achieved, place a piece of parchment paper on top and use a heavy and flat object to help you press down firmly. This will help it even out.

4. At this point, the oven should be fully heated. Place the baking dish in the oven and cook the dough for 15 minutes. At this time, increase the temperature to 375 degrees and cook for 5 minutes more. This allows for the crust to cook separately from the rest of the ingredients, which is necessary to achieve a solid, flaky crust. However, keep an eye on the crust to ensure that you do not overcook it. You want the edges to be a golden brown and not too dark. Take out of the oven so it can cool.

5. While this is happening, take a small saucepan and add in the cornstarch, sugar, a pinch of salt, and almond milk. Add in the almond milk while you are whisking in order to stop the mixture from clumping. Mix this until it is completely combined with as few lumps as possible. After this, put the saucepan on medium heat until it begins to boil, all the while stirring to ensure that nothing is sticking and burning. At this

point, reduce the heat and allow it to simmer for 5 minutes. Make sure to be constantly scraping the sides and the bottom of the pan.

6. After this time, it should take on a bouncy like quality, much like jello or pudding. Take it off the heat and drizzle in the vanilla extract. Stir in completely and let it cool for 8-10 minutes. After this, transfer to a glass bowl and cover with plastic. Be sure to cover this completely as it will ruin the consistency if it comes in contact with air for too long. Put in the refrigerator for 2 and a half hours.

7. While you are waiting for this stage to complete, put take a medium sized glass bowl and put it into the freezer. Take the can of coconut cream, open it carefully, and remove the solid portions. Leave the liquid behind, as this is not needed in this recipe. Be sure to not shake the can while opening it, as this would mix the contents. That is, you need the liquid and the solid to be seperated. Put the solids into the glass bowl from the freezer.

8. With an electric mixer, mix the coconut solids until it begins to resemble whipped cream. This should take 1-2 minutes. After this, add in a few drops of the vanilla extract and about 2 tablespoons of the powdered sugar. Whip this again for another 2 minutes, until it becomes even more light. Then, put it in the refrigerator to chill.

9. After the filling has been in the refrigerator for 2 ½ hours, it should be entirely cooled. At this point, you can add it to the whipped coconut cream. There is no need to whip these together, just lightly combine them. Once this is complete, put them back in the refrigerator to stay cool.

10. Now, take a banana and slice into thin slices. Put these slices at the bottom of the crust. Put the filling mixture on top and make sure to smooth it with a spoon to ensure that it is evenly distributed. Cover with plastic, put it in the refrigerator, and let it set for over 4 hours. If you have time, it is better to let it set even longer, perhaps overnight.

11. You can serve this like any other pie, in that it is best to cut it into triangles slices. You can also top this with other types of fruit, more bananas, powdered sugar, etc.

Notes: This is a fairly easy dessert that does not require any baking, so the options to include other ingredients is fairly wide open. For example, instead of bananas, you can try raspberries, blueberries, blackberries, etc. You can also try incorporating cocoa powder into the filling to give a different flavor profile. Perhaps you can even try experimenting with different fruit nectars or concentrates, instead of using sugar. For example, you can drizzle agave nectar over the top, instead of finishing the pie with powdered sugar. You could also try blueberry syrup, raspberry syrup, or any other type of fruit based syrup. For vegans that are willing to eat honey, this would also be a good opportunity to use it.

Vegan Brownies

Ingredients List:

- 2 cups of walnuts, without the shell
- 1 ½ cups of almonds
- 2 cups of dates, dry without the pits
- 1 cup of cocoa powder, unsweetened is preferred
- 2 tablespoons of cacao nibs
- 1/4 teaspoon of salt
- 1/4 cup of non dairy milk, unflavored almond is preferred
- 1 cup of dark chocolate, find the kind without dairy
- 2 tablespoons of coconut oil
- ½ cup of powdered sugar

Steps:

1. Take a food processor and put the walnuts and the almonds inside. Process these until they are broken down into small pieces. After this, add in the cacao powder and a pinch of the salt. Combine these together until all the ingredients are

evenly distributed. Take the mixture out and place in a bowl. Set this aside for later.

2. Take the same food processor, and put the dates in. Process the dates until they are broken down into small pieces. At this point, you want to slowly add in the nut and cocoa mixture back into the food processor to combine with the dates. Do this a little at a time, as it will thicken up quickly, causing the ingredients to clump and not be evenly distributed.

3. Keep processing the mixture until it begins to form a dough like consistency. If the dough does not hold together well, add in more dates. This dough will form the base of the brownie mixture.

4. After this take a small baking tray with high sides and add the dough. Place a piece of parchment paper on top and find something heavy and flat for you to push down with. This will help flatten the dough and make sure that it is the same thickness everywhere. When finished take the walnuts and the cacao nibs and sprinkle them across the top evenly. Once these are on top, put the parchment paper back on and push down once again. This will push everything into the dough. However, be sure to save some of the cacao nibs for the topping.

5. Next, remove the dough from the dish. At this point, you can use your hands to push and squeeze the shape, if you desire them to be a bit thicker or smaller. After this, put them back into the pan and place into the freezer for 15-20 minutes, thus allowing them to firm up significantly. Once this is done, you can remove them a cut them into squares.

6. Before serving, you can make the ganache, which is a delicious topping for your brownies. The first step of this is to put the almond milk into a small bowl and microwave until it becomes warm. This should take less than a minute. You can also do this in a saucepan on the stove if you desire.

7. Once it is brought up to the desired temperature, begin to add in cacao nibs and stir in until fully dissolved. After this, add in a pinch of salt and continue to stir to ensure that it is not

sticking to the bottom or to the sides. Then, put in the coconut oil, again stirring until it is fully incorporated.

8. Put this mixture into the refrigerator for 10-15 minutes. This will give it a chance to thicken, turning into a syrup like consistency. When this has been achieved, take it out of the refrigerator and add in powdered sugar. Be sure to add this in slowly, as pouring it all in at once will result in clumping. Stir this in until everything is fully incorporated. At this point, you can begin stirring and beating the mixture vigorously. This gives the mixture a fluffier consistency.

9. After this, apply this topping to the brownies. How you do this is up to you. You can apply an even glaze across the top or you can simply drizzle it on in whatever pattern that you would like. You can also add extra walnuts to top if you want.

Notes: This is a great recipe that offers a lot of extra options if you cannot find certain ingredients or if you do not like something. For example, if you do not like walnuts, then you can substitute almonds instead. For an extra flavor dimension, you can try toasting the nuts before adding them to the top or into the mixture. To do this, simply take a dry non stick frying pan on medium heat and place the chopped nuts inside. Slowly move the pan around until the nuts are golden brown. You can also try chopped pistachio nuts, which will certainly give it a unique flavor. Also, if you cannot find dates, these can be substituted for figs, which are essentially the same. However, his will give it a slightly different taste. Furthermore, these brownies would go well with chopped fruit on top. Try putting strawberry or kiwi slices on top before serving. It is up to you which extra ingredients you add, but keep in mind that dates and figs have a very specific flavor profile. Therefore, some foods do not pair well with them, even though they might seem like they would.